Thomas Dancer

A Brief History of the Late Expedition Against Fort San Juan, So Far As It Relates to the Diseases of the Troops

Together with some observations on climate, infection and contagion; and

several of the endemial complaints of the West-Indies

Thomas Dancer

A Brief History of the Late Expedition Against Fort San Juan, So Far As It Relates to the Diseases of the Troops
Together with some observations on climate, infection and contagion; and several of the endemial complaints of the West-Indies

ISBN/EAN: 9783337317294

Printed in Europe, USA, Canada, Australia, Japan

Cover: Foto ©ninafisch / pixelio.de

More available books at **www.hansebooks.com**

A BRIEF HISTORY

OF THE

LATE EXPEDITION

AGAINST

FORT SAN JUAN,

SO FAR AS IT RELATES TO

THE DISEASES OF THE TROOPS:

TOGETHER WITH

SOME OBSERVATIONS ON CLIMATE, INFECTION AND CONTAGION;

AND SEVERAL OF THE

Endemial Complaints of the *West-Indies.*

By THOMAS DANCER, M. D.
PHYSICIAN TO THE TROOPS ON THAT SERVICE.

KINGSTON.

Printed by D. DOUGLASS & W. AIKMAN, and sold by them at the Royal Gazette Printing-Office, and at WM. AIKMAN's Shop in Kingston; by ALEXANDER AIKMAN, at the Printing-Office in Spanish-Town; and by JAMES FANNIN, Printer in Montego-Bay.

MDCCLXXXI.

TO

HIS EXCELLENCY

GENERAL DALLING,

GOVERNOUR of the Island of JAMAICA,

CAPTAIN-GENERAL, VICE-ADMIRAL,

AND CHANCELLOR OF THE SAME,

AND THE TERRITORIES THEREON DEPENDING:

THE FOLLOWING PAGES,

On the HISTORY and DISEASES of the
LATE EXPEDITION againſt FORT SAN JUAN,

ARE HUMBLY INCRIBED,

BY

HIS EXCELLENCY's
MOST OBEDIENT AND DEVOTED SERVANT,

THE AUTHOR.

INTRODUCTION.

IT is not the defign of the author of the following pages to write a full hiftory of the expedition: The object and conduct of that fervice, with every thing refpecting the military department, he is totally unqualified to judge of, and will therefore no further enter into his confiderations, than as they are connected with his defign; which is to explain the caufes of that general ficknefs and mortality that prevailed among the troops; and to make a few obfervations on fome of their difeafes. The ficknefs or health of troops, however, depends fo much on their fituation and movements, that he will be obliged to take fome account of thefe; and it is therefore propofed to give firft a fuccinct hiftory or journal of the campaign, and then to make fome general remarks on the endemial difeafes of foldiers in the Weft-Indies.

CORRIGENDA.

Page 19—line 14—Read, *many of which*, instead of, *which many*, &c. Ibid. line 10—Dele, *being*. Ibid.—line 15—For, *made*, read, *were*. Ibid.—line 19—Dele, the comma after the word *hospital*.

Page 31—line 12—For *infected*, read *affected*.

Page 34—line 6—For *fatid*, read *fætid*.

Page 40—line 1—For *from*, read *by*.

Page 44—line 6—For *was*, read *were*.

Page 56—line 9—For *evacuations*, read *evacuants*.

Page 51—line 7—For *for*, read *and that*.

A BRIEF

HISTORY

OF THE

LATE EXPEDITION, &c.

THE circumstances of time, command, number of troops, and their embarkation to go upon a SECRET EXPEDITION; from its having been framed in this country, but more especially from its fatal issue, and the private misfortune it has occasioned to many, in the loss of friends; are so well known, and will have so lasting an impression, that it will be here quite unnecessary to mention them. It will be sufficient, for the sake of more general information, just to observe, that in the beginning of the year 1780, a small army, consisting of about two hundred Regulars, of the 60th and 79th regiments, one hundred men of Major DAL-RYMPLE's Loyal Irish corps, and two hundred Jamaica Volunteers,

Volunteers, were sent by his Excellency GENERAL DAL-
LING, under the command of Colonel JOHN POLSON, up-
on a secret Expedition against some part of the SPANISH
territories in South America.----This little army having
embarked on board several transports, we set sail from
Port-Royal on the 3d of February, under convoy of the
Hinchinbrooke frigate, and directed our course first for the
Musquito Shore.

ALTHOUGH the autumn and winter of 1779 had been
in Jamaica very sickly, and many of the troops had died;
it must be observed, that those sent upon service being all
selected, were at the time of our departure in general good
health, and continued so during the voyage:---two men
only died on the passage, both of them convalescents from
long fevers; one of them, having a return of fever, with
symptoms of immediate putrefaction, died in a very short
time; the other, being very weakly, and not able to scuffle
amongst the men upon deck, remained constantly in his
birth, and, from lying always on the same side, got a mortification in the hip, which, notwithstanding the instant
and free use of bark, and wine, &c. soon carried him off.
This case deserves to be noted, because such accidents are
very liable to happen to men in that situation, and, in the
bad air of a ship's hold, will always prove very dangerous,
if not incurable.

THE

THE Penelope tranfport having run aground, a poor man of the Voluntcers on that occafion had the misfortune to have his fkull dangeroufly fractured; the fracture ran acrofs both the fagittal and lambdoidal futures; and, by means of the trepan, a number of fragments of the os occiputis were extracted, and a confiderable part of the dura mater, & finus longitudinalis, expofed.---The operation was performed under every poffible circumftance of difadvantage; but, by the fingular care and attention of Mr. Watfon, furgeon of the corps, he recovered, and continued pretty well for fome time, 'till, being feized with the flux, he afterwards died.

ON the 14th of February, we arrived at Cape Gratias à Dios, where the foldiers being difembarked, were encamped on a large plain, about a mile from the fea, called Wank's Savanna. The foil of this plain is very fwampy, affording water at only a foot or two below the furface.---Between this favanna and the fea runs a pretty large river, called alfo Wank's, furrounded by Scot's grafs, mangroves, and other woods, to a confiderable diftance, fo as to generate an unwholefome air, and to feclude from the camp the falutiferous fea breezes. Our men muft have inevitably become very fickly, had they remained long in this place; but befides that our ftay was fhort, the feafon was then fair: the water, which contained a very ftrong chalybeate impregnation, might perhaps have been alfo of ufe to
them,

them, by carrying off the bile, and by a tonic power in bracing up the folids. To many indeed the water gave a diarrhœa, which, notwithftanding the means made ufe of for reftraining it, perfifted while they continued to drink it.

Whilst at this place, we had a few intermittents, but our whole number in the hofpital did not exceed thirty, till the arrival of Captain Dalrymple and Mr. Schomberg from Black River, with a party of men of the 79th regiment, who were almoft all of them in a moft deplorable condition, from old intermittents, dropfy, and flux: we had alfo a few other fluxes, which, upon enquiry, I found had been brought from Jamaica, and two of the number died.

On the 10th of March, our troops being reimbarked, we in a few days took our departure from Cape Gratios à Dios, and, after anchoring at feveral places on the Mufquito Shore, to rendezvous with the Indians who were to proceed with us on the Expedition, we arrived on the 24th of March at the river San Juan; our men in general good health, and in great fpirits, from the idea of being fo near to the deftined fervice.

About two hundred regulars, being difembarked from the tranfports, with the neceffary equipment of ammuni-

tion

tion and ftores, proceeded immediately up the river with the Indians in their feveral crafts, a particular kind of boats fo called: It being then the latter end of the dry feafon, the river contained very little water, and was full of fhoals and fandy beaches, which rendered our paffage exceedingly difficult: The men were frequently obliged to quit the boats, and unite their moft ftrenuous exertions in getting them along through a number of fhallow channels, previoufly explored by Indians, fent before for that purpofe. This labour continued for feveral days after we left the mouth of the river, till we arrived in deeper water, when we made a quicker progrefs: but our men were much expofed to injury, from the fun's rays beating violently upon them for feven or eight hours every day, befides a ftill more intenfe heat reflected from the many naked fhoals, covered with a whitifh fand, which rendered the air fometimes intolerable. This violent infolation during the day, was followed by as dangerous an expofition to the heavy dews at night; and it was furprifing that the men continued fo well; for as yet we had but few, and thofe trifling, complaints.

I cannot omit the occafion of doing our Indians the juftice to mention their fpirited exertions and perfeverance, in the arduous enterprife of rowing up the boats fuch a length of way againft the many obftacles we met with: we were no lefs obftructed by currents, than by fhoals;

B and

and the rapids or falls occafioned us ftill greater difficulty;
but the Indians have a fingular addrefs on thefe occafions,
and I cannot help thinking that we were greatly indebted
to them: for the foldiery, partly from ignorance in thofe
matters, and partly from that indolence which was the
natural effect of their fituation, were frequently of very
little ufe: The ftrefs of this bufinefs, therefore, lay chiefly
upon the former; and this accounts for their complaints
coming earlier on, than thofe of the foldiery.---It muft be
obferved, that the Indians are not a hardy race, efpecially the
true unmixed ABORIGINES of the country. The Cape Indians, who have an admixture of negro blood, feem to be
fuperior to thofe mentioned ‡, both in the powers of mind
and body; they are in general taller, more mufcular, and
have an afpect expreffive of a greater fhare of intelligence:
However we explain it, the fact was, that they did not fall
ill fo foon as the others. Thofe Indians who could be fpar-
ed from their boats, proceeded on before us, and were no
lefs active than dexterous in procuring us plenty of game,
and fifh, which contributed not a little to the fupport of
our mens' health, under that fhare of fatigue they fuftained,
and the expofition they were fubject to.

ON the 9th of April, we arrived at a little ifland in the
river, called St. Bartholomew, which was fortified by a
fmall horfe-fhoe battery, mounting nine or ten fwivels,
and

‡ *Vide* in the Abbé REYNAL's Hiftory of the Indies an account of this.

and defended by a garrifon of twelve or eighteen men.---
This ifland was poffeffed as a *look-out*, but being previoufly
reconnoitered, Captain DESPARD, with a party of men,
was fent through the woods to furprife them: After a few
fhots, they endeavoured to fly; but were prevented in their
retreat by the Indians, who were pofted higher up for that
purpofe.----On this occafion, only two men received any
hurt: one was fhot in the abdomen; but the ball having
paffed through his cartridge-box, did not penetrate the
cavity:---the other had three fingers of one hand very
much fhattered, but foon recovered the ufe of them.

A MUCH more melancholy accident happened to one of
the men on their march through the woods: a fnake, hang-
ing from the bough of a tree, bit him as he paffed along,
juft under the orbit of the left eye, from which he felt fuch
an intenfe pain, that he was unable to proceed; and when
a meffenger was fent to him a few hours afterwards, he was
found dead, with all the fymptoms of putrefaction; a yellownefs, and fwelling over his whole body; and the eye,
near to which he was bitten, all diffolved.

THE fnakes of this country are very numerous, and of
feveral kinds *, moft of which are efteemed highly poifonous,

* *PISO* reckons about twenty different fpecies in BRASIL; which I fhould
fuppofe are moft of them alfo inhabitants of this part of the coaft.

THIS part of Natural Hiftory, though in the higheft degree interefting to
the human fpecies, has not been fufficiently cultivated: We are ftill, in a
great

ous, but not equally fo: The Indians feem to dread moft
a fmall one, called by them *tomagafs*.---The moft ordinary
kind, called (from the manner in which it is marked) the
Barber's Pole, is not fo virulent as the former.   The common remedy, and the only one that I could learn of, is the
antidote, or ✝ *calabafh coccoon*, as it is called here, and I
                                                      prefume

great meafure, unacquainted with thefe noxious animals; and it is an object
that claims the attention of natural inquirers, to inveftigate more particularly the fpecies and diftinctions of thefe reptiles, together with the proper
antidotes againft their feveral poifons.——I fhall here fubjoin a fketch of the
general arrangement of the ferpent tribe; for which I am obliged to the Re-
verend Mr. ROBERTS, a gentleman completely verfant in all the departments
of natural knowledge.

 THE celebrated *LINNÆUS* has arranged the ferpents into fix *genera*, viz.
1. CROTALUS, which is diftinguifhed by having the fcuta of the abdomen
    and tail terminated by a rattle: This genus contains five fpecies, all
    venomous.
2. BOA, which is known by having the fcuta of the abdomen and tail termi-
    nated without the rattle: It contains three fpecies, which are all inof-
    fenfive.
3. COLUBER, of which he enumerates ninety-feven fpecies, fixteen of them
    are poifonous:—This genus is known by the abdomen being covered
    with a fcutum, and the tail with fcales.
4. ANGUIS, having both the abdomen and tail covered with fcales.—There
    are fixteen fpecies of this genus, but none of them poifonous.
5. AMPHISBÆNA, containing only two fpecies, both harmlefs:—The abdo-
    men and tail of the animals of this genus are marked with rings.
6. CÆCILIA, containing two fpecies, both harmlefs;—they are known by
    their being covered with wrinkles.
Note, Thofe ferpents that are venomous are furnifhed with fangs, fomewhat
refembling the tufks of a boar:—they are moveable, and inferted in the
upper jaw.

 ✝ This plant is beft defcribed by BROWN, in his Natural Hiftory of *Jamaica*,
under the name of *fevilla*: the feeds or kernels of this plant are frequently
ufed by the negroes in a fpiritous infufion, which makes a ftrong bitter, and
                                                      a large

presume the same as ULLOA calls the *habilla*, or *snake bean*. This, as well as other antidotes that have been celebrated, may be possessed of some virtues, but are not of that established efficacy to be with safety depended upon : it may, therefore, not be improper, in this place, to suggest the means to be pursued under such a misfortune.----Suppose any one so unhappy as to be wounded by any of these poisonous reptiles, the most (if not the only) effectual remedy, is, an immediate excision of the part; or, if that should not be practicable, to scarify the parts about the wound, and, by suction, or cupping glasses, if they can be procured, to extract the virus before it passes forward into the blood. ---It is to be observed, that, notwithstanding the direful effect which those poisons exhibit when they enter the system, that they have no action or influence in the mouth or stomach; and the wound may therefore be sucked with great safety by another person ‡.-----A burning-hot iron

C applied

a large dose proves both emetic and cathartic :—it is called by the negroes the *antidote*, as they entertain the same notion with the Indians, of its alexipharmic virtues.—There is no doubt of its being a very useful medicine, and worthy to be introduced into the officinal list, if the seeds did not lose their qualities by keeping: but how far it may be justly considered as either a general or specific antidote, it is impossible to determine, as we have no other evidences than the testimony of the Indians and negroes, who, in their opinions concerning the medicinal efficacy of plants, &c. are chiefly guided by superstition.——These seeds being of a very oily nature, the negroes frequently burn them as lights; and Mr. ROBERTS has discovered a mode of making from them a most excellent kind of candle, not inferior even to wax, or *spermaceti*.

‡ The MARSI and PSYLLI, two ancient nations, were possessed of this secret.—It is probably by absorption that the snake stones act, if they have any action at all.

applied to the part, may be ufed in the place of excifion, but perhaps with a lefs certain effect: befides, it is feldom that fuch a means is at hand on fuch an emergency, and there is no time for delay; for if once the poifon is abforbed, and has paffed onward into the circulating fluids, local remedies can have no effect. The ufe of olive or common falad oil in the bite of the viper ||, is very univerfally known, and fhould not be omitted to be applied to the parts, after what has been recommended. Emetic and fweating medicines have alfo been efteemed ufeful, and fhould be employed: refpecting the latter, they fhould be continued fo as to prolong the fweat for a confiderable time.

On April the 11th, we came in fight of the caftle of San Juan, and on the 13th the fiege commenced, which, with fo fmall an army, was not carried on without much fatigue and difficulty.---Added to the hard labour of throwing up batteries, and the common military duty of maintaining a number of guards and pofts, the men had to tranfport all the ammunition and ftores, by a very bad road, through the back woods, from the landing place two or three miles below the caftle.

For fome time, the animation excited by profpects of victory and fuccefs, enabled our men to refift every impreffion from the fatigue and labour they underwent: but at length the Seafons, or bad weather, fetting in, the whole army,

|| *Vide* MEAD on Poifons.

army, both the foldiers and the Indians, began to fall fick, efpecially the latter, who fuffered more from their own inhumanity, and want of care towards each other, than from any other caufe; as, though abfolute fatalifts, it is a kind of cuftom amongft them, never to regard or pay any attention to their fick, further than to place them under fome tree or hut, and giving them water.----Such was the indolence, obftinacy, and infatuation of this people, that no reprefentation or remonftrance that was made to them, could prevail on them to unite their endeavours for the building a houfe or hut for the reception and accommodation of their fick friends, who, lying under fevers and fluxes, expofed to all the inclemencies of the weather, derived little advantage from the affiftance of medicine, and many of them, as might be expected, died.---The diffatisfaction and defertion of thefe allies, foon after the furrender of the caftle, delivered me from any further trouble concerning them: and I have only to add refpecting them, that I remarked nothing very peculiar in their complaints, except that they were in general more inflammatory.

THE hills which our army occupied, afforded fo many favourable and fecure pofts, that our men were very little expofed, and met with very few accidents; two or three only were killed, and not above nine or ten wounded.---In the number of thefe, we had one cafe which was very remarkable, and I fhall therefore give the hiftory of it.---A
failor

failor of the *Hinchinbrooke* being a little intoxicated, purfued
down the hill, under the enemy's fire, a hog that he had endeavoured to kill.   He received two or three fhot; but one
of them took a very extraordinary courfe, which I believe
moft people would think fatal.   The ball entered by the
groin, and traverfing the pelvis, came out through the
glutei mufcles, near to the knob of the ifchium.   The
fpermatic cord was very much contufed, and inflammation
was come on before I faw him; fo that, although I fufpect-
ed great danger would arife from a fubfequent mortification
of the tefticle, followed perhaps by a fatal hemorrhagy from
the veffels, I could not then make ufe of either the knife, or
the needle.   As to the injury of the vifcera, I could not then
judge, but it did not afterwards appear, either by his ftools
or urine, that they had fuffered any accident.   The gan-
grene and hemorrhagy, as was apprehended, came on, and
threatened great danger ; but the latter being reftrained by
ftyptics, the only means that in that cafe could be employed, he took large quantities of bark and wine, along with
the beft nourifhment that could be procured for him ; and
he recovered.

THE Caftle having furrendered on the 24th of April,
we hoped that our victory would furnifh us, not only with
accommodations, but with many ufeful fupplies, that might
tend, in fome degree, to ftop our increafing ficknefs; but,
alas ! the wretched ftate of the garrifon, provided with nothing

thing that could lend either them or us the leaft comfort; and the inconvenient ftructure of the place, which was worfe than any prifon, and, as one would fuppofe, calculated only for the purpofe of breeding infection, difappointed us in thofe flattering expectations. Our men, therefore, now falling down in great numbers, added to all their other misfortunes, had no proper hofpital for receiving them;-the wretched houfes or fheds to which we were obliged to give that name, being from their fituation not only fo nigh the river, but under the Caftle-hill, and totally fecluded from the fea-breezes;-from the dirt and filth furrounding them, confifting chiefly of femi-putrid fkins, yielding a moft intolerable ftench;-from the infufficiency of the roofs, which many of them kept out very little rain; made them, I will not fay merely an improper hofpital, but a certain grave to almoft all who entered them.---Add to what has been mentioned, the circumftances of a moft unhealthy climate; the Seafons, or inceffant rains, alternating with the moft extreme heats; the want of hofpital, neceffaries, and accommodations, and fometimes of medicines, and it will not be wondered at, either that the troops became fo fickly, or that fo few recovered *.

D

MANY

* THE hiftory of all Weft-Indian armaments unhappily correfpond too much with that we are now giving of the Expedition againft Fort *San Juan.* I need not mention the fatal affair at *Bocca Chica*, fo pathetically related by THOMSON, in his SEASONS.——

When o'er this world, by equinoctial rains
Flooded immenfe, looks out the joylefs fun,
And draws the copious fteam: from fwampy fens,

Where

MANY of the afore-mentioned circumſtances may ſeem, to thoſe unacquainted with the particulars of the ſervice, to have been remediable: The queſtion may, in the firſt place, be aſked, Why, as there was no building fitted for the

> Where putrefaction into life ferments,
> And breathes deſtructive myriads; or from woods,
> impenetrable ſhades, receſſes foul,
> In vapours rank and blue corruption wrapt,
> Whoſe gloomy horrors yet no deſperate foot
> Has ever dar'd to pierce; then, waſteful, forth
> Walks the dire Power of peſtilent diſeaſe.
> A thouſand hideous fiends her courſe attend,
> Sick Nature blaſting, and to heartleſs woe,
> And feeble deſolation, caſting down
> The towering hopes and all the pride of Man.
> Such as of late, at Carthagena quench'd
> The Britiſh fire. You, gallant VERNON, ſaw
> The miſerable ſcene; you, pitying, ſaw
> To infant-weakneſs ſunk the warrior's arm;
> Saw the deep-racking pang, the ghaſtly form,
> The lip pale-quivering, and the beamleſs eye
> No more with ardour bright: you heard the groans
> Of agonizing ſhips, from ſhore to ſhore:
> Heard, nightly plung'd amid the ſullen waves,
> The frequent corſe; while on each other fix'd,
> In ſad preſage, the blank aſſiſtants ſeem'd,
> Silent, to aſk, whom Fate would next demand?

——Nor is the mortality amongſt our brave troops at the *Havannah* yet forgotten:—The affecting letter of an officer on that ſervice, which ſo well deſcribes our unhappy ſituation at *San Juan's*, I ſhall here take the liberty to quote from Doctor LIND:—" I think myſelf extremely happy in being among " the number of the living, conſidering the deplorable condition we are now " in:—Out of 100 men which I landed, I have only now 33 left in my com- " pany. Our regiment has loſt 8 officers, and 500 men. Out of 17 battali- " ons, we cannot muſter 600 men fit for duty:—they died chiefly of *intermit- " tent fevers* and *fluxes*."——

——The late dreadful mortality of the troops at *Lucia*, as well as at other parts of *America*, ſerve to evince the inſalubrity of theſe climates, and the difficulty attending all military operations in this part of the world.

the purpofes of an hofpital, was not one erected? To this I muſt anſwer, that although the unhealthineſs of theſe houſes were repreſented to the Commander-in-chief, and his orders obtained for building a proper hofpital, theſe orders could never be carried into execution; the ſickneſs becoming ſo general, that there was neither artificer to work, or ſoldier to aſſiſt him: Neceſſity then compelled us to make uſe of places that became a ſource of contagion, and precipitated thoſe who went into them out of the world. ---As to hofpital accommodations, ſuch as bedding, and the ſeveral articles of ſugar, oatmeal, &c. we had them in an abundant quantity, but not at our hofpital, where they were wanted: there being not a ſufficient number of craft for tranſporting the ammunition and ſtores up the river; a certain quantity only of each could be put on board, which in many cafes was not competent to the exigencies of the ſervice; and the ſickneſs increaſing, rendered our future ſupplies from the tranſports ſtill more precarious. So general was the illneſs at this time, and ever afterwards, that, independent of the few who were well enough to do garriſon duty, we had not orderly men ſufficient to aſſiſt the ſick.---The deplorable ſituation of ſuch a number of men labouring under ſuch complaints, and lying in ſuch places, without the requiſite aſſiſtances, and the uſe of the neceſ-ſary means for preſerving † cleanlineſs, and a ſweet air, can

be

---

† Nihil tamen æque morborum phalanges in caſtra invehere poſſe credide-rim, quam caſtrorum ſordes et neglectam munditiem: Divino edicto olim Iſ-raelitis interdicibantur, ne intra caſtra alienas fæces auderent deponere;— ſed, &c.———Vide *Rammazini de morbis artificum.* DEUTERONOMY.

be eafily judged of: The fevers and fluxes, therefore, that in the beginning were dependent on climate, &c. and affecting only individuals, became afterwards evidently contagious, and feized almoft every one who came within the infection ‡: few of thofe who arrived in health (though this number was very fmall) efcaped for many days the reigning malady.

THE weather clearing up for a fhort time, gave us fanguine hopes that our men would now recover, but moft of them relapfed again upon the return of the rains; and at length, in the month of September, the army, fo much exhaufted by ficknefs, returned down the river, leaving only a proper garrifon at the Caftle.   The ufe of a better nourifhment, which the harbour afforded, particularly fifh and turtle, it was hoped might be of great ufe to convalefcents; but the contrary event happened.   The inordinate appetite which attended people reduced by long ficknefs, being too freely indulged, was productive either of indigeftion and crudities in the *primæ viæ*, or a too fudden and general impletion, which proved very injurious to them; and a better food, inftead of promoting their health, ferved rather to haften their exit.

THE

‡ Authors are not generally agreed, whether *intermittents* are properly contagious:—*Cleghorn, Lettfom,* &c. think they are infectious:—the dyfentery and remittent fever, into which they are frequently changed, are unqueftionably fo.

THE ficknefs and mortality of the troops ftill continuing, I prefume it was thought neceffary to decline the further profecution of that fervice; at leaft till a proper reinforcement fhould arrive, and the feafons become more favourable. The remainder of the army, therefore, embarked for Bluefields, an Englifh fettlement about twenty leagues to the northward; but the exhaufted and debilitated ftate which moft of the men were in at the time, rendered the fituation and air of a fhip's hold very mortal to them, and a great number of them died on their paffage.

A total lofs of my own health obliged me about this time to apply for leave of abfence; and I have therefore nothing further to add on the fubject of the campaign, but to acknowledge, not in my own name only, but in that of many, the affiduous and humane attention of our Commander-in-Chief * to every thing that could tend to the recovery of the fick, and health of the army: but all the offices of the kindeft humanity, all the efforts of the beft informed judgment, neither the benevolence of the heart, nor the fkill of the mind, could avail againft the united oppofition of fo many formidable enemies †.

---

* Colonel KEMBLE of the 1ft Battalion of the 60th Regiment.

† Among thefe, the *climate* muft be confidered as the principal one. The country is overfpread with wood: on the fides of the river are numberlefs ftinking marfhes; and the rains fall in torrents through the greater part of the year.——From the month of April, when the caftle furrendered, till October, when the army returned down the river, and for fome time after this, the rains continued, with now and then a lucid interval of a few days, to fall in prodigious quantities, and fometimes with the moft dreadful thunder ftorms. *Carpenter's river*, or *Matina*, the neareft fettlement on that part of the coaft, is reckoned by the Spaniards another *Rio Morte*. The torrents of rain to which Carthagena is fubject, fall, according to REYNAL, from the month of May till November.——*Vide Hift. Ind*. and *Wafer's account of Darien*.

E

OBSERVATIONS

o n

Climate, Infection, and Contagion.

OBSERVATIONS ON CLIMATE, &c.

CLIMATE.

THE effects of different climates in producing difeafes of a different nature and tendency, has been
remarked in all the ages of mankind, and treated
of with great judgment, even by HIPPOCRATES, the fa-
ther and founder of phyfic.----" Quicunque artem medi-
" cam, inquit, integri confequi volet, hæc faciat opportet.
" Primo quidem temporum anni, rationem habeat; nulla
" enim in re fimilia funt fed multum differunt; tum ipfa
" ad invicem, tum in propriis permutationibus, deinde
" etiam ventos calidos et frigidos, qui unicuique regioni
" funt peculiares," &c.----The obfervations of authors on
this fubject amount to this, that in cold climates, people
have a greater degree of tone, or that their fibres are more
tenfe and rigid; and that, in confequence of this, they are
more fubject to inflammatory complaints, or fuch difeafes
as, in their nature and cure, require a treatment, as blood-
letting, and other evacuations, whofe effects are, to dimi-

F   nifh

nifh this tone or tenfion of the fibres; while, on the other
hand, from the natural property of heat *, people in all
warm climates become very much relaxed, and are fubject
to difeafes, not of the aforementioned inflammatory kind, but
to thofe of a putrid tendency +.----The difeafes, then, of
cold climates are principally, inflammatory fevers, coughs,
confumption, rheumatifm, pleurify, &c.; but, in warm
ones, the fevers are of the bilious, remittent kind ‡, frequently becoming putrid: and thefe are not only the moft
ordinary kinds of fever, but the difeafes which moft ordi-
narily happen: For it may be obferved, that although we
cannot, in the Weft Indies, boaft of equal health with
thofe in northern climates, we can yet aver, that we are
fubject to fewer difeafes.----Difeafes of the inflammatory
clafs, as well as of every other kind, do indeed occur in
warm climates, but not fo frequently, or with fo much
violence. Upon the whole, the catalogue of maladies in
the Weft Indies is much lefs than in Europe; but then the
fevers,

* Calor fi nimius eft, corpus effeminat, nervos emollit, ftomachum folvit
obnoxium morbis peftilentibus corpus efficit.——CELSUS *de Medicina.*

Calor acris vi fua relaxante corpus debilitat.—Syftematis, tum fenfibilita-
tem, tum mobilitatem auget.—Fluidorum tenuitatem et acrimoniam auget.
Diff. Med. BOWDLERI.

† WILSON on the influence of climate.

‡ The remitting fever is truly one of the fixed, regular epidemics (*endemics*)
of the ifland of Jamaica, and is more or lefs prevalent in the months of October, November, and December. I look upon it to be the fame as that of
Minorca, Sumatra, Java, and of other parts of the Eaft and Weft Indies.
NASMYTH *in* LIND's *Eff. &c.*

fevers, which conftitute the greater part of this catalogue, are, from the effects of climate, and the difference of conftitution, of a much more dangerous tendency.

WHATEVER influence *heat* * may have, either upon the folids or fluids in the human body, in altering their natural condition, we know, that it is greatly increafed by the union of moifture. People, during the hotteft feafons, and in the hotteft climates †, often preferve a moderate fhare of health; but, after heavy falls of rain, they in general become fickly.---This is a fact well known by all thofe who have inhabited the Weft Indies, and other warm climates.

IT is not, however, either heat or moifture, fimply confidered, that produce fevers ‡, but, along with thefe, fenfible
                                                                qualities

---

* Heat alone has certainly the effects before-mentioned: but the judicious Doctor NASMYTH, who to the many opportunities he had of determining this queftion, j ined a very particular attention, has obferved, " That the incon- " veniences and difeafes arifing from mere heat, are far lefs confiderable than " has been imagined."———*Vide* LIND's *Effay*, &c. *p.* 56.

† The temperature of the air in South Carolina and Georgia, in fummer time, according to the experiments of Mr. ELLIS, much exceeds that of the human body; yet the inhabitants bear it with health and unconcern.
                                                          GOLDSMITH's *Nat. Philof.*
Some curious experiments have lately fhewn, that the human body is capable of fuftaining a furprifing degree of heat, without any confiderable annoyance of the functions.———*Vide Philofoph. Tranfact.*

‡ *Calores* fane fummi fine febre. Peftis enim fub maximis caloribus extinguitur. Nec *humore* abundantes, illico febris eft. Æftivas imbres fore ubique fa'ubres; civitates quoque falubres juxta flumina fitæ, &c.
                                                     Drummond de feb. ardend. &c.

qualities of the air; and, originating from them, there is
another caufe of difeafe, which, though of a latent nature,
acts upon the human body with much more force and activity: This caufe is, the poifonous effluvia or miafmata a-
rifing from the ground, in all woody and marfhy fituations,
particularly in warm feafons, and in warm climates. || The
endemical or prevailing difeafes of people inhabiting all
fuch foils, efpecially during fuch feafons, prove beyond a
doubt the exiftence of thefe miafmata †; and it is more
than probable, that all fevers of the intermittent and remittent kind, depend conftantly upon fuch a caufe.---Heat
and moifture may feparately have their effects upon the human body; but it is their influence, when united, that raifes
thefe noxious exhalations, which produce the fevers, and
other endemial difeafes of warm climates. It is heat acting
upon moifture that generates thefe miafmata; and therefore
it is in autumn, after the heavy rains which fall in that
feafon, that fuch difeafes moft prevail. Rain alone, or inundations of water, feem not, without the affiftant energy
of heat, to have any effect: for, it is not till after thefe
have paffed off, and the humid furface of the ground be-

comes

|| In regionibus feptentrionalibus, ubi frigora intenfa et continua funt, fe-
bres intermittentes nunquam incidere; contra in plagis meridonalibus, ubi
calores magni funt praec'pue in aeftate et autunno graffari obfervavit *Lancijius
de noxiis Palud. effluv. lib. 1. c. 5.—Grieve de feb. int.*

In locis paluftribus, in aquae ftagnantis vicinio, juxta lacus fordentes foffaq.
febres intermittentes endemicae funt.

† CULLEN'*s firft lines Pr. Phyf.*

comes expofed to the fun's action, that this procefs, fo fatal to the human fpecies, begins * : then the infection in all fuch places rages; and it frequently happens, that the inhabitants are univerfally affected.---Many fuch unhealthy fituations are there in this ifland, which being, on account of a greater degree of moifture, more fertile, are more cultivated and inhabited, but not without fhewing effects that prove the truth of what has been obferved †.

THE influence of thefe miafmata feem to be in proportion to the proximity of their fource; for, according as people inhabit places that are near to, or far off from the marfhes, they are more or lefs infected.----The fame circumftance alfo occafions a variation in the type of fever; the nearer the patient refides to the infectious fomes, the lefs his fever is difpofed to intermit, and is more commonly a quotidian; when living at a little greater diftance, the fever is generally a tertian; and when ftill more remote, a quartan.----It is alfo worthy of remark, that the action of

G   thefe

* PROSP. ALPINUS *de morbis Ægyptiorum*, mentions, that during the inundations of the Nile, people are very healthy; but as foon as the inundation ceafes, and the muddy furface of the earth is fubjected to the influence of the fun, then the epidemical difeafes of that country begin.——This fact, long taken notice of, is recently confirmed, in the account Mr. ROLLO has given of the ficknefs of the troops at St. Lucia.

Vide LANCISIUS *de nox Palud. effluv.* SENAC *de recondit. feb. nat. p.* 35.

† Many of thefe places are taken notice of by LIND, in his " *Difeafes of hot* " *climates,*" particularly Greewich, which proved fo unhealthy, that it was found neceffary to remove the naval hofpital to Port-Royal.

thefe effluvia feem to be confined within very narrow limits, except when tranfported by winds to a greater diftance.--- Many curious facts prove inconteftibly the truth of thefe obfervations *; and a proper regard being had to them, may be the prefervation of innumerable lives.

Such is the operation of heat and moifture in producing febrile contagion; but there is ftill to be taken notice of, another fpecies of contagion, which, for the fake of diftinction, is more ftrictly and properly fo called :---This is, the effluvia of the human body, or the odour arifing from other fubftances that have been impregnated with it. The human body, confined long together within its own atmofphere, and not having its perfpirable matter carried off from it, can, as we know·from a great many inftances, produce a contagion capable of affecting others, though the perfon himfelf remains in health † : but fuch a contagion is much more likely to arife from the body when difeafed : And in this manner the plague, fmall-pox, and nervous and putrid fevers, are produced and propagated. ‡ To what circumftances

* Lind's Eff. &c.——Rollo on the difeafes of the army at Lucia.—— Bowdler Diff. de Intermitt.

† This has been evidenced in a number of cafes, particularly in the well-known one of the prifoners at the Old Bailey.

‡ Piso denies the influence of contagion in hot climates, even in the dyfentery.—" Hæc excretio, inquit ille, licet pari vehementia per omnes Indias fæviat, nunquam tamen in Brafilia morbi epidemici inftar, graffatum alioque per

ftances it may be owing, whether to a greater degree of
heat in volatilating and fubtilizing matters more, or to the
conftant breezes, which prevent any ftagnation, I know
not; but fo it happens, that contagion operates much lefs
in warm, than in the temperate climates. This is particu
larly obfervable in fevers, which are feldom contagious,
not even the highly putrid one, called the *yellow* fever [*].
In the cafe of fluxes, however, where the contagious matter
is more predominant, it acts more generally, and produces
a difeafe fatally infectious. There is fo near an affinity between the intermittent and dyfentery, that they frequently
interchange and alternate with each other, fo as to give a
fufpicion of their arifing from a common caufe: in both
cafes, there is a copious fecretion of bile, which, in con-
currence with other caufes, may fometimes determine the
difeafe in one way, and fometimes in another; producing at
one

per contagionem migraffe conftat."——*Vide* Pison *de utriufq. Indiæ re medica
& naturali.*——Bontius, who treats of the difeafes of the Eaft Indies, is
of a different opinion, and has evinced, by feveral examples taken from a number of others, that epidemical difeafes occur there, with all their proper fymptoms, &c. fpread by contagion.——*Vide* Bontius *de epidem. et contag. in
Indicis, morbis.*

[*] Hilary's difeafes of Barbadoes.
   It is very fingular, that the putrid yellow fever, though never contagious in
the Weft-Indies, is yet extremely fo (according to *Lining*) in Carolina:—*Vide
Ff. Phyf. & Lit.* Nay, further, it would feem, that although the contagion
does not operate in the Weft Indies, there is nevertbelefs one produced; for
fome wearing apparel, belonging to a patient who died of the yellow fever,
being fent from Jamaica to his friends in America, they fatally infected them
with the fame difeafe.——*Vide* Lind's *Ff. &c.*

one time an intermittent, and at another a dyfentery †. In whatever manner the latter difeafe may be produced, among individuals, it no fooner arifes than a fatal contagion is generated, which univerfally infects thofe who come within the fphere of its influence, and chiefly by means of the fatid ftools ‖, that feem in this diforder to conftitute a dangerous fomes.----By a *fomes* is meant, any thing which, by accumulating and retaining the infectious matter, renders it more active and virulent : Thus, not only the ftools of the difeafed, but their apparel, the bedding and furniture, with the very walls of the apartment in which they lie, are contaminated, and acquire the power of affecting others, even more than the emanations proceeding directly from the human body.

THE nature of contagion is altogether infcrutable, but the properties of it, which have been enumerated, are confirmed ‡, by a number of melancholy, and not lefs curious incidents.

† PRINGLE's difeafes of the army.

‖ Some fecretions are more apt to convey infection than others ; the ftools feem moft commonly to communicate the taint ; next to thefe the breath, and laftly, the effluvia of the body.——LIND's Eſſ. &c.

ALEXANDER is of opinion, that marfh miafmata are not putrefcent, but antifeptic ; and he infers, therefore they are not hurtful : but the conclufion is both againft reafon and fact.——He is alfo of opinion, that the faces never generate contagion, though he admits that they are very effectual in propagating it.

‡ Of twenty-three men who were employed in repairing fome old tents that had belonged to fick people, only fix furvived the infection which they imbibed.——Pringle.

incidents. Caufes that are not vifible, or very obvious, are not apt to ftrike mankind in general with much force; and it is difficult to perfuade many people of the exiftence or efficacy of fuch latent powers: But there is the moft abfolute demonftration to be given of what has been mentioned, and a knowledge of thefe circumftances will tend, in many cafes, particularly in camps, towards the prevention of the moft fatal diforders.

In the preceding fheets I have fhewn, that all the caufes of a bad climate, infection, contagion, &c. prevailed in an eminent degree at SAN JUAN's; and that, along with thefe, every thing confpired to give them their full force and activity; I fhall now, therefore, proceed to confider the difeafes themfelves, fo produced, and to make fome obfervations on the principal complaints of the Weft Indies.

H   O F

Five or fix people died in fucceffion, who were put into the apartment of one who had died of a bad fever, notwithftanding the utmoft pains being taken to purify it.—It was at laft found neceffary to plane the floor, and new-plafter or white-wafh the room.———*Brockleſby*.

A whole nation of Indians in Nova Scotia, called *Mifmachs*, were deftroyed by fome infected blankets which they had picked up at *Chebreto*, after the departure of the Duc d'Anville's fquadron.———LIND's *Eſſ*. *Traite de malad, des gens de mer, par* POISSONIERE.

OF THE FEVERS, &c.

IT is not my prefent defign, to attempt a full treatife on WEST INDIAN difeafes:--having fo little to add to what the many excellent authors on this fubject have already delivered, I fhould efteem it an undertaking equally vain and ufelefs: I mean, therefore, to confine myfelf to a few of the moft important circumftances, relating to thofe diforders which prevailed among our troops on the late EXPEDITION:--Thefe were chiefly, as we have before feen in the narrative of the campaign, intermittent and remittent fevers, and the dyfentery or bloody-flux, the conftant endemics of every part of the Weft-Indies, particularly of the moft unhealthy parts, and during the unhealthy or rainy feafons. Thefe complaints, though not effentially differing from thofe of the fame kind in Europe, are neverthelefs attended with fome peculiarities, and require fome variation in practice.

A redundant fecretion of bile ever attends this clafs of difeafes in every climate, but remarkably fo in all hot ones; and has been always fuppofed to have a great influence upon the diforder in its progrefs. It is alfo fuppofed, that the bile is frequently vitiated in its quality, and being reabforbed into the fyftem, carries along with it a putrid ferment, that

causes

caufes an immediate and total diffolution of the fluids, as in the yellow fever.

This preternatural fecretion of bile in hot climates, which has been obferved even from the time of *Hippocrates* and the commencement of phyfic, is with great difficulty accounted for, and I fhall not attempt it *: It is fufficient that we know the fact; and I fhall therefore confine my enquiries to the effects of it, and confider only what influence the quantity and ftate of the bile may have in producing fevers, &c. or in changing their proper nature. From the conftancy of this fymptom in moft fevers, the ancients were of opinion that they arofe from this fource:--Bile was confidered by them as the immediate caufe of fever; and this opinion has almoft univerfally obtained, through all fucceeding ages to the prefent time †.

An enquiry into the truth of this doctrine, is a fubject worthy of a fuller difcuffion than can be here admitted of; but I fhall ftate a few circumftances relating to it.----Bilious congeftions, or bile on the ftomach, is the almoft univerfal and conftant complaint of the inhabitants of hot countries, even in a ftate of health, or when they labour under no other difeafe; and all the effects that generally arife from it, when other caufes do not coincide, is an impaired appetite,

a little

* *See* M'Lurg's *Experiments on the Bile.*
  Experiences chimiques fur la bile de l'homme, par Monf. Cadet.
† Mead's *Monita & Præcepta.*----Sinac *de record. feb. nat.*

a little naufea, principally in the morning before the tak‑
ing in of frefh aliment; vitiated digeftion; now and then
a diarrhœa; or fometimes, on the contrary, a coftivenefs of
the bowels ‡. Thefe complaints take place in proportion
to the excefs of bile on the ftomach, and are fometimes in
a confiderable degree; but ftill they fubfift without fever,
--It is plain, therefore, that a redundant fecretion of bile,
cannot be confidered as a direct and immediate caufe of fe‑
ver, although, by diminifhing the tone of the ftomach, it
may difpofe the body to be more forcibly acted upon by the
proper febrile caufes : And hence we fee, that people who
have recovered from a fever, are exceedingly liable to relapfe,
from this difordered ftate of the ftomach.

IT may be further obferved, that bile is often not only
very innocent in the ftomach, but even, when abforbed and
mixed with the fluids, produces none of thofe dire effects
of which it has been accufed :---jaundice is not attended
with fever, nor does it feem to give any difpofition to‑
wards it ‖.

                                                              IF

‡ HIBERDINE obferves, that the bile, being a ufeful fecretion, may, like
the faliva, be fometimes increafed in its quantity, without any detriment to
the health.——It is not likely (he adds) that the health fhould depend on any
precife quantity of bile, for fometimes there is none poured out for many days;
and, vice verfa, the healthieft perfon may, by going on board a fhip, become
in the fpace of a few minutes deluged with bile, without feeling any confe‑
quences after he goes on fhore.——Med. Tranfact. vol. 2.

‖ Sed fi febris caufa fit bilis, quandem peculiarem eamq. infolitam fibi ipfa
adificat neceffe eft; nam exundat fæpiffime Ano et Cato abfq. ulla febris in‑
faltu; nec vero in eam magis proni funt qui ictero laborant.
                                                  SENAC de recend. feb. nat.

IF the bile fhould ever be the caufe of fever, it muft be owing to fome foreign and acquired property, not to an excefs of the natural fecretion; for bile, as we have feen, is not only a fluid abfolutely neceffary to the functions of the ftomach, but, when in its natural ftate, appears to be of a very innocent quality, producing no immediate bad effects though mixed with all the other fluids of the body. It is, however, fuppofed, that the bile is of a very putrefcent nature *, and fufceptible of a high degree of acrimony; which being diffufed over the fyftem, produces in certain fevers a total diffolution of the fluids.----All the writers who have treated of that fpecies of putrid remittent, called the yellow fever, have affigned for the caufe of it, a corrupted putrid bile abforbed into the fyftem †: But, with all deference to the many excellent authors who have entertained this opinion, I muft beg leave to ftate fome difficulties attending it.

MANY alterations happen in the ftate of the bile, as well as in its quantity, without any confiderable effect upon the health. The change of the bile which is moft obvious, and which moft commonly occurs, is that of acidity. In fome cafes it has proved fo corrofive, that when vomited it has excoriated the mouth, and deftroyed the enamel of the teeth; but this has happened without any other confequence

I   or

* From the experiments of Sir JOHN PRINGLE, it would feem that this notion is in a great meafure ill founded.

† HILARY on the difeafes of Barbadoes.

or effect upon the general health : what has been so often affirmed, of the putrid nature of it under some fevers, is totally devoid of proof, and the opinion has probably been drawn merely from some unusual appearances in it, from an admixture of other matters *.

ANOTHER circumstance of difficulty respecting this theory, is, that as dissections have never shewn any obstruction of the gall-duct, as in the case of jaundice, how should the bile be more than usual absorbed ? † It is even allowed, by those who adopt this notion, that the icterical colour of the body, or yellow suffusion under the skin, in some bad fevers, proceeds more from a putrid dissolution of the blood and exudation of the serum, than to a proper jaundice or admixture of bile with the fluids ‡.---There is no doubt but the notion of these fevers originating from the bile, took its rise from the yellow tincture of the skin; but this we see is owing to another cause : we see, that the bile is not absorbed in an uncommon quantity, nor does it appear certainly, that the bile suffers any material change from its natural state; why then should the bile be suspected on this occasion ?---But, admitting every thing that has been said concerning the bile, we may still doubt whether the effect is not taken for the cause. An increased secretion of bile, and a vitiated state of it, may attend fevers, without being
the

* HEBERDEN in the Medic. Transact.
  MONRO's Diseases of the Army.
† LIND's Diseases of hot Climates.

the caufe of them: The bile will be fubject to alterations fimilar to thofe which happen in all the other fluids, and may verge towards putrefaction; but this is not obfervable in the incipient ftate of the difeafe; it is only in the progrefs of it, and when a general putrefcence comes to prevail.

FROM what has been faid, is it not more probable that the nature and termination of thefe fevers depend either on fome peculiarity in the contagion, or on fome particular cir- cumftances in the fyftem, as a high degree of phlogiftic diathefis, a fcorbutic tendency, &c.?---Many facts relat- ing to the yellow fever feem to confirm this opinion, for it attacks chiefly thofe of a fanguine and plethoric temperament, and efpecially thofe coming newly from Eu- rope, or a cold climate. Further, the practice of blood- letting, fo much decried in the Weft-Indies and other hot climates, has in this cafe been found of the utmoft utility. HILARY * employed the lancet very freely in the beginning of this fever, and repeated it even after fome appearance of diffolution in the fluids: whence the neceffity or propriety of this, but from the circumftances fuggefted? It is there- fore fufficiently clear, that it is not the ftate of the bile, but the condition of the habit, which gives this putrid type to the fevers of hot climates.

BEFORE I difmifs this fubject, I muft beg leave to men- tion another opinion that obtains pretty generally refpecting
the

* *See* Difeafes of *Barbadoes*.

the bile; which is, that the use of certain foods and liquors
have the effect of increasing and vitiating this secretion.---
The possibility of this cannot be denied, but there are no
facts to ascertain it †.   The disagreement of certain foods,
nausea, and consequent vomiting of bile, is no proof of it,
for the bile discharged might have been before present in the
stomach.----Malt liquors are more especially criminated with
this quality; but the disagreement of them may perhaps be
rather owing to their viscidity, rendering them of difficult
digestion in weak stomachs.   The nausea they in such cases excite, may also beget a more plentiful effusion of bile
into the stomach; but I am inclined to suppose, that when
drank only in quantities proportioned to the digestive powers, they have no such effects as has been imagined, and e-
ven prove, in many instances, highly medicinal.

HAVING digressed so far, to examine into the question
concerning the influence of the bile in generating fevers,
or in determining their particular nature and tendency, I
shall now go on to make some more particular observations
on the several species of fever incident to our army.

INTER-

---

† It has been imagined by some physicians, that aliments differ in their effects upon the bile; some increasing its acrimony, &c.—but what they have
said seems to me loose and inaccurate.——Whether there are any such sub-
stances that have peculiar properties with respect to the bile, I dare not determine.   CULLEN's Mat. Medica.

INTERMITTENT FEVER.

OUR fevers were principally of the intermittent kind, efpecially upon the commencement of our ficknefs; and being attended with all the ufual fymptoms, I fhall not detain my reader by the hiftory of what is fo univerfally underftood. Not to dwell upon minutiæ, or matters that are uninterefting, I fhall omit every thing that experience did not lead us to pay a particular attention to.----In the firft place, I have to obferve, that our intermittents were chiefly of the quotidian or tertian form, efpecially the latter:----quartans we had no example of that I can remember. This type of an intermittent is every where lefs frequent than the preceding, and in the Weft Indies is, I believe, rarely met with, unlefs among children; and in their cafe proves very obftinate, continuing fometimes for years, in fpite of every means that can be employed. The attack generally came on after fome unufual degree of fatigue, or expofition to the bad weather, with all the ordinary fymptoms of this kind of fever, purfuing its progrefs through the feveral ftages of the cold, hot, and fweating fits: In the quotidians, which partook more of the nature of the remittent, the cold fit was not always fo confiderable, but in the tertians was long protracted, and very fevere; fo that it was fometimes with great difficulty that a patient was conducted through it *.

K   A

* Authors are difagreed with refpect to the moft dangerous period of the paroxyfm. It is the prevailing opinion, that the cold fit is commonly moft
fatal;

A JAUNDICE, or univerfal yellownefs, now and then came on, which, though not fymptomatic of any putrefcence, was generally a bad prognoftic, as hardly any fuch cafes ultimately recovered †.

Obftructions of the vifcera, particularly of the fpleen ‡, was the confequence of this fever, when long continued; but the frequent termination of it into a remittent or dyfentery, prevented thefe from happening very often.

THE ordinary eruption of puftules about the lips and noftrils, or boils breaking out over the furface of the body, generally indicated a crifis or folution of the fever, though the patient was not afterwards fecure from a relapfe.

As I recollect no other circumftances of peculiarity in the hiftory of our intermittents, I fhall proceed to make fome obfervations on the treatment of them.

TREATMENT

fatal; but others affirm, that patients dying with an intermittent, generally go off during the hot fit :—it was the cold fit that proved fatal with us.

                        See MORTON, LIND, &c.

  † This was inftanced in the cafe of a very worthy gentleman, Captain BERTRAND of the *Jamaica Volunteers*, who died foon after this appearance came on; as alfo in the much lamented Mr. GASCOIGNE of the LXXIXth regiment, who, after going through every ftage of the epidemic, the intermittent, remittent, and dyfentery, at laft yielded to the common fate.

  ‡ The liver, according to almoft all authors, is the vifcus moft generally affected (*vide* SENAC): but I do not remember to have feen in our hofpitals any cafe of protuberance and hardnefs on the right fide, or in the hepatic region: the fpleen feems to be moft commonly and fooneft affected.

TREATMENT OF INTERMITTENTS.

In Europe it is of great importance to diftinguifh between intermittents of the different feafons: The vernal
are in general more eafily removed, and blood-letting proves
a principal means of cure *; but in the autumnal agues,
this remedy is ufed with greater caution.

THE fame caution is required in all hot climates, on account of the putrefcent difpofition of the fluids: but perhaps this may have been carried too far: Inftead of totally relinquifhing the lancet, as is the practice of fome
phyficians †, it may be only neceffary to ufe it more fpar-
ingly. There are few fevers in which it is not, during
fome periods of the difeafe, more or lefs admiffible ‡: but
ftrict regard muft be always had to the fymptoms and conftitution of the patient, as thefe only can determine the
proper quantity of blood to be drawn: this muft be always
lefs in hot than in cold climates, though it is not eafy to
eftablifh any certain proportion. The fymptoms principally
indicating venæfection in intermittents, efpecially in hot
climates,

---

* SYDENHAM.

† The Englifh Phyficians in the Weft-Indies are exceedingly cautious in
bleeding; while the French, Spaniards, and Portuguefe practife it very freely,
as in Europe.———LIND's Eff. &c.
'The Abbe RAYNAL fays, 'That fo rapid is the progrefs of nature in the hot
climates, that it is frequently neceffary to bleed fifteen or eighteen times in
the firft twenty-four hours:—He very properly fubjoins, that the prieft, law-
yer, and phyfician are generally called at the fame time.———Hift. of Indies.

‡ CLEGHORN found, that blood-letting was not only admiffible, but even
neceffary, in the intermittents at Minorca.

climates, are local affections, as pleurify, pains in the head,
&c. which often accompany them : but even here, local
bleeding may prove more beneficial.   The tendency of intermittents to change into remittents of a putrid kind, or
into dyfentery, fhould infpire us with ftill greater timidity
refpecting the ufe of the lancet, and on this account blood-
letting was very feldom ufed in the intermittents which
the troops laboured under at SAN JUAN's.---There are,
however, fome cafes, in which bleeding may prevent the
fever from becoming remittent, and even change it to a
regular intermittent; but thefe depend on a phlogiftic
diathefis, and feldom occur in hot countries, unlefs a-
mong negroes.   The moft eligible period for ufing the
lancet, when it is required, is during the hot fit, when all
the inflammatory fymptoms are moft exafperated; but as
this is a remedy fo feldom judged neceffary, let us go on to
confider thofe which are efteemed of more importance.---
Among thefe, *vomits*, from their general utility, and the
time at which they are commonly given, in the firft place
claim our attention.

THE ftate of the *primæ viæ* in fevers, renders the ufe of
emetics abfolutely neceffary for the purpofes of evacuation.
The bile, and other fecretions, together with the aliment-
ary contents of the ftomach, under the increafed heat, and
other circumftances in the fyftem depending on fever, may
be changed in their nature, and rendered highly acrimonious, if not putrid, fo as not only to give in the beginning
a great

à great degree of ſtimulus, but to make a deleterious im-
preſſion on the brain and nervous ſyſtem.

However important it may be to procure a free diſcharge
from the ſtomach, this is not the chief action of emetics;
they are poſſeſſed of virtues that render them ſtill more beneficial; they cauſe a determination to the ſurface of the
body, and thereby remove the ſpaſm on the ſmall veſſels;
or, to ſpeak more intelligibly to a reader unacquainted with
medical ſcience, they produce a ſweat, and a ſolution of fever.---This effect of emetics has been long known *, though
not ſufficiently attended to till of late: SYDENHAM, who
conceived of emetics as evacuants only, ſtood ſurpriſed at
their good effects, even when they produced but little vomiting: Their operation in this way is, however, now ſufficiently underſtood, and the practice of giving them in ſmall
doſes †, to procure nauſea only, is become univerſal, after
having firſt evacuated the ſtomach by a free and full diſcharge.---The utility of this practice is ſo well confirmed
by general experience, that, like all other eſtabliſhed remedies, it is liable to abuſe: It is ſometimes perhaps carried
too far, and in that caſe it proves extremely debilitating;
beſides, the antimonial preparations employed for this pur-
poſe are too irritating for ſome ſtomachs, and much miſ-
chief will accrue where they are not judiciouſly doſed:
The clamour againſt exceſſive bleeding is outrageous, but

L

hardly

---

* See WEPFER.
† CULLEN's Firſt Lines.———LETTSOME on Fevers. &c.

hardly any one thinks of the poffibility of vomiting a man to death.---There is, therefore, fome nicety in the adminiftration of emetics, which we found by experience in the fevers at SAN JUAN's; for the ftomachs of the patients were frequently fo irritable, as not to bear them. In this cafe, more advantage is derived from lenient *cathartics*, given in fmall and repeated dofes, till the defired effect is produced.

I SHALL not enter into a general difquifition concerning the ufe of cathartics in intermittents; but it may be proper to obferve, that exceffive purging, like all other evacuations, is in hot climates very debilitating; for which reafon, the neutral falts, cr. tartar, tamarinds, manna, &c. have been long preferred by good practitioners, to others of a more heating and acrid quality *. I beg leave alfo to fuggeft, that, when given in fmall dofes, they may poffibly act upon the fkin in a way fimilar to emetics; at leaft, the ufe of them in this manner is preferable to that of giving them in full dofes, as they agree better with the ftomach, and procure ultimately more copious evacuation, with lefs ftimulus and agitation.

THE Englifh HIPPOCRATES (SYDENHAM) firft recommended the ufe of opium in intermittent fevers, a practice that has been fince found, by the experience of others, and

particularly

---

* In regionibus calidis, cathartica refrigerantia, fructus, fales neutri, &c. præfcribenda quia valde irritabilis eft tubus inteftinalis.

BRANDRETH *de feb. intermit.*

particularly the immortal Lind, to be of the higheft utility.---It has been obferved, that opium given before the
acceffion of the paroxyfm, will fometimes ftop it *; but
the more eligible and approved method, is to give it at the
end of the cold fit; and the effects produced by it are, an
abatement of all the fymptoms during the hot fit, a more
plentiful fweat, and a more complete intermiffion †.---
Thefe good effects I have feen follow from the ufe of opium
very frequently; and one would be inclined to fuppofe, that
whatever advantages attend the practice in cold climates,
much greater would follow from it in warm ones.

Omitting the confideration of feveral other remedies,
I fhall conclude what I have to fay on intermittents, by a
few thoughts on

The Bark.

So much has been written on the virtues of this medicine, and to remove every objection to the ufe of it, that
it is fcarcely poffible to add any thing on the fubject: I
fhall therefore take notice only of a few circumftances relating to its adminiftration.---Much has been faid by many
excellent writers ‡ againft the ufe of the bark previous to
evacuations,

* Berryat.——Gregory's Prælectiones.
† Hoc (fc. Opium) tempore caloris exhibitum, vim febris frangit, duratio-
nemque contrahit, capitis dolorem delirium et id genus alia rævenit.
                                             Brandreth.——Lind.
‡ Van Swieten, &c. &c. &c.

evacuations, or the removal of bilious congeftions in the
primæ viæ; but in the fevers of hot climates, there is frequently no time allowed for thefe: fuch is the force and
violence of the fymptoms, that if the bark is not given immediately *, the patient infallibly falls a victim to delay.
In fuch cafes, therefore, thefe objections muft be fet afide;
and experience has amply evinced, that they are without
foundation †. It is, notwithftanding, proper to join evacuations with the bark, when you cannot ufe them previous to it; and by this means the objections, if of any force,
are in fome degree removed.

ANOTHER difficulty attending the adminiftration of the
bark, is the irritable condition of the patient's ftomach,
which renders him infufceptible of a proper dofe, and
fometimes hinders him from taking it at all.----I fhall fay
nothing of the well-known methods of combining it with
opium, aromatics, &c. but, as thefe will not always fuc-
ceed, the only remaining alternative is that of clyfters, fo-
mentation, &c. thefe are often efficacious: But, as I cannot
quit my view of military hofpitals, I muft obferve, that thefe
modes of exhibiting it are in an army frequently impracti-
cable. I take the liberty, therefore, to propofe the method
of fprinkling it plentifully over the furface of the body;
if there be any moifture on the fkin, a great part of it will
adhere,

* CLARKE's Difeafes of long Voyages.——CLEGHORN's Dif. of Minorca.
† MONRO's Difeafes of the Army.——CLEGHORN's Difeafes of Minorca.
It was the cuftom of thefe practitioners, to give the bark with purging falts, &c.

adhere, and a fufficient degree of abforption take place, to render it beneficial. The efficacy of the bark jacket * has been long known, and I can therefore fee no objection to this practice, but the great confumption of bark it might occafion. To this it may be anfwered, that it is only recommended, where it cannot be more effectually employed in fmaller quantities; for life is more eftimable than a few pounds of bark.

EXPERIENCE has lately determined, that the efficacy of the bark in a great meafure depends upon the time of giving it: it was originally given during the paroxyfm, but it was foon found to be much fafer and better in the intermiffion : ftill it is enquired, at what time of the apyrexia ought it to be given? The idea of its efficacy depending on its antifeptic † properties, &c: has induced moft practitioners to throw it in as early as poffible after the intermiffion commences : but, confidering fever according to the CULLENIAN theory, as arifing from debility, and that the bark operates as a tonic ‡, the proper time of giving it is confequently at that period when the atonia begins to take place, viz. juft before the paroxyfm. Fact has demonftrated this beyond a doubt ‖; and it is a maxim of great

M   importance

---

* MORTON.   † Sir JOHN PRINGLE.   ‡ CULLEN's. Mat. Med.
‖ Doctor HOME produces fome experiments to the contrary of this; but it is probable that they were not inftituted with fufficient care :—However that might be, two or three exceptions cannot invalidate a general fact.———See , Clinical Obfervat. and Exper.

importance to be attended to in the adminiſtration of this uſeful medicine.---The patient, however, is not always able to take the bark in conſiderable doſes; and it is therefore requiſite, in order that a due quantity of it may be taken, to anticipate the return of the atonia:--In the quotidian *, it is neceſſary to give it almoſt as ſoon as the intermiſſion comes on; but in the tertian, &c. there can be no occaſion to nauſeate and haraſs the patient by hourly doſes of a diſagreeable medicine during the whole interval, eſpecially when we conſider, that, by previouſly loading the ſtomach, we are prevented from giving it in full doſes, at the time when it is capable of producing the greateſt effect.

THE virtues of the bark, like thoſe of every other medicine, are tranſitory; and, to perpetuate its good effects, it is neceſſary to continue its uſe, or repeat it from time to time: when this is neglected, fevers that were ſtopped are liable to return †, and, from the debility already occaſioned by previous ſickneſs, they often put on a bad appearance, and become more unmanageable.

I HAVE only one more circumſtance to add, viz. that as bitters of every kind have, in ſome degree, the ſame powers

as

* CULLEN's Materia Medica.

† I has been long a received opinion, that the moon has a great influence upon the plants and animals of our earth; and a very ingenious writer has endeavoured to confirm this opinion by a variety of obſervations:—He ſays, that at the full of the moon, fevers are more diſpoſed to return, and that the bark ſhould be repeated in particular at that time.

                    Vide WILSON on the influence of climate.

as the bark, they may be fometimes vicarious to it :---In a fcarcity of bark, I found, that an infufion of camomile flowers, made in a flight decoction of the bark, anfwered almoft as well as the bark itfelf. MEAD's powder ‡ has alfo, on fome occafions, proved more beneficial than other bitters, or than even the bark.

REMITTENT FEVER.

THIS fever, in its mode of attack, and in moft circum-ftances, greatly refembles the intermittent; but having only an abatement of its fymptoms, or no perfect apyrexia ||, it partakes more of a continued nature, and therefore has in it more danger.---The fymptoms are likewife in this fever more violent; at leaft the patient becomes, in the progrefs of the difeafe, fooner exhaufted, and the fluids tend more quickly to putrefaction. A univerfal yellownefs fometimes comes on, conftituting what is then called the yellow fever; concerning which I have before had occafion to make fome remarks: and as we had few, if any, examples of that particular fpecies of remittent, I fhall not now repeat what was before mentioned. A yellow fuffufion did indeed attend many of our fevers, both remittent and intermittent, but this was evidently icteritious, and not proceeding from a diffolution of the fluids : A degree of putrefaction alfo came on in the latter ftage of the fevers, but feldom with thofe haemorrhages, and other direful fymptoms which accompany the remittent called the yellow fever.

AMIDST

‡ This confifts of camomile flowers and alum. || Intermiffion.

AMIDST such a multitude of sick as we had at the castle
of San Juan, in the number of which were almost all the Fa-
culty themselves, it was impossible to be very minute in
observations on particular cases. To shew an equal humanity towards all, a partial neglect towards individuals was
indispensible †; and therefore, an infinity of circumstances
in the practice of physic might have escaped my attention :
as for example, I was never able to determine any thing
precisely concerning the critical days; the existence of which
in these fevers has been so often asserted and denied.

TREATMENT.] The intermittent and remittent, being
so nearly allied as to their symptoms, cannot differ much in
their cure : but as in the remittent there is greater danger,
there is also required more vigilance and circumspection.
This is particularly necessary with regard to bleeding and
the use of vomits. Venæsection may be hazardous in intermittents, but is in general much more so here, from the
quicker progress of the fluids towards putrefaction.---Pro-
blematical, however, as it may seem, there are certain cases
which require bleeding on this very account. In plethoric
patients, and where the symptoms run very high, the early
and discreet use of the lancet will promise more advantage
in mitigating the violent reaction or ardency of fever, than
it can possibly do hurt by debilitating the patient : the putrefaction,

† Mais il arrive souvent que le nombre des malades est si grand dans une
armee, & qu'ils sont dispersees en tant d'endroits differens qu'il est impossible
que les medicins se portent partout & puissent donner leurs soins a chacun d'eux.

trefaction, inftead of being accelerated, is by this means retarded. It is only in this way that we can account for the fuccefsful effects of bleeding, even in the yellow fever *.

GREAT caution is alfo neceffary in the exhibition of vomits; for it fometimes happens, that the ftomach is fo much weakened by fpontaneous efforts, and becomes fo irritable, that the ufe of them is highly dangerous.---Infufions of camomile flowers and opiates are found the beft means of allaying thefe efforts, and to prepare the ftomach for receiving gentle *laxatives*: Thefe are to be given as foon as poffible, to carry off the bilious colluvies in the firft paffages; but thofe of the moft agreeable kind are to be chofen, as it is neceffary to give them in repeated dofes. An obftinate fpafm on fome part of the bowels, feems to be fometimes induced by their acrimonious contents, which lenient medicines are infufficient to remove; but, on the other hand, draftic ones would be highly improper,---In thefe cafes, I have found a few grains of calomel combined with opium the moft efficacious means of procuring the needful evacuations. Great attention is required to regulate thefe as foon as they come on, encouraging or reftraining the ftools according to circumftances and the ftrength of the patient. Cordials are frequently neceffary, to fupport the vis vitæ while this operation is going on, and to hinder it from proceeding too far, which may produce a fatal debility. The bark likewife is to be given as early as poffible, or as foon

N   as

* *Vide* HILARY's Difeafes of *Barbadoes*.

as the ſtomach, being cleared of its irritating contents, is
rendered capable of bearing it, either in ſubſtance, or in
any other form.---The danger that ſometimes reſults from
delay, has been before mentioned with reſpect to intermittents, but here it is ſtill greater; and if we are determined
to proceed in the ſlow methodical way, of always vomiting,
purging, &c. and then waiting for obvious remiſſions, the
death of the patient will frequently diſappoint our expectations *.---The ſerpentary has been found in general a very
uſeful addition to the bark, and an excellent ſuccedaneum
where the bark could not be internally made uſe of.   Hilary, in the putrid yellow fever, found it impoſſible to
give the bark + in any form; and therefore, of neceſſity,
depended on the ſerpentary, which he ſays proved no leſs
ſucceſsful.

Amongst the other cordials neceſſary to ſupport the
ſtrength of the patient, wine is the moſt important, and
chiefly deſerves our conſideration ‡; but the adminiſtration

of

---

* In locis aduſtioribus, autumnale tempore paroxyſmis ſane paucis, quam-
plurimum periclitantur, febricitantes; hic igitur ubi primum poteſt, quam-
vis obſcuriores ſint remiſſiones, cortex adhibendus eſt Peruvianus.—*Brandreth.*
See alſo Clarke's *Diſ. long Voyages* —Percival's *Eſſays.*—*Medic. Tranſact.*—
Huck in Pringle.—Cullen's *Firſt Lines.*

† Percival ſuppoſes, that this diſagreement of the bark was owing to
the ſavor which ariſes from an admixture of it with the bile; and as acids
have the effect of neutralizing the bile, he thinks, that by a combination of
theſe with the bark, it will be rendered leſs diſagreeable to the ſtomach.

‡ In febribus malignis, vino nihil datur excellentius; in iis morbis reſtau-
rare vires; ſpiritus erigere; circulum ſanguinis liberum reducere tranſpira-

of it is attended with some difficulties. The nature of the delirium muſt be carefully diſtinguiſhed ; and the doſe relative to the ſymptoms and conſtitution of the patient, muſt alſo, by careful obſervation, be found out before we proceed in the free uſe of this beſt of all cordials. For want of ſuch a judicious diſcrimination, much hurt may be ſometimes done by a medicine otherwiſe calculated to produce the moſt happy effects. The pulſe affords the trueſt indication for the continuance of it : if from being feeble and quick, it becomes fuller and ſlower, eſpecially if the patient, being delirious, becomes more coherent or diſpoſed to eaſy ſleep, there is the fulleſt proof of its benign influence ; but when it is given improperly, the patient, if not delirious before, frequently becomes ſo, or ſtill more diſturbed ; and his pulſe is at the ſame time not only more full, but much accelerated.

HAVING already too much exceeded the bounds of this ſubject, I have only to obſerve further, that reſpecting the choice of wines to be given in fevers, claret is the one moſt generally uſeful, having the greateſt cordial effects, with the leaſt ſtimulus ; but when the vis vitæ is much depreſſed, and a greater ſtimulus required, Madeira wine will be preferable, as it contains a greater portion of ardent ſpirit †.

DYSENTERY.

tionem movere ; expedit. et in ee verſatur omnis alexipharmacorum virtus.-
HOFFM. Op. tit. v. p. 353.———Vide GILCHRIST, HUXHAM, &c.

† Vide NEWMAN on Wines.

DYSENTERY.

THIS difeafe, in certain feafons of the year, and in certain fituations in the Weft-Indies, is commonly endemic, and, from its contagious nature, often becomes e-pidemical, efpecially in towns, camps, and hofpitals, where it proves of all others the moft dreadful diftemper.----The ftools of the difeafed, which are always extremely fætid, feem to be, as has been before obferved, the principal fo-mes and means of infection ‡ ; and by this, as well as feve-ral other circumftances, the dyfentery is eafily diftinguifhed from diarrhæa.----Of the dyfentery alfo there are feveral fpecies, which in practice it is requifite to attend to : but it is the epidemic contagious dyfentery that is here the fubject of confideration. This is the general companion or follower of intermittent fevers, attacking people during the fame feafon of the year, and fometimes alternating with them : Thence the opinion, that the two difeafes fpring from one common parent, which has been generally fuppofed a putrefcent bile ‖ .----That bile is not the caufe of fevers, has been already demonftrated * ; but ftill it is not impoffible, that a certain ftate of bile, produced by fe-

ver,

‡ Cette maladie infecte bientot toute une armee: les exhalaitons putrides des matieres fæcales infectent furtout les foldats fains lorfqu'ils fe feivent des memes latrines.———V. Swisten.

‖ It is reafonable to believe, that the dyfentery is owing to a caufe little different from that which produces bilious fevers : The ancients attributed both to an abounding and corrupted bile.———Pringle *Dif. Army.*—Zim-merman, p. 23.   * See page 37, &c.

ver, may have a confiderable influence in bringing on this complaint. However certain that may be, it is evident that a fpecific contagion is afterwards generated; and is it not therefore more probable, that fever has only the effect of fubjecting the patient to the influence of a new infection? It is perhaps impoffible to determine this queftion, but there is an obvious, though inexplicable union between the two difeafes.

To avoid as much as poffible a beaten tract, and to keep this publication within its intended limits, I muft omit the hiftorical detail of this, as I have done of the diforders before treated of, and proceed to a few remarks on the method of cure, which will comprehend every thing effential that my experience qualifies me to take notice of.

THE treatment of the dyfentery was formerly but very ill underftood; and, notwithftanding a better method of cure has been of late difcovered, the difeafe may ftill, in fome degree, be confidered as the *opprobrium medicorum:* at leaft, the efforts of phyficians to prevent the fpreading of this infection, particularly in camps and hofpitals, have in a great meafure been unavailing. The feveral means by which the progrefs of this difeafe is moft effectually reftrained, have been amply treated of by all the writers on camp difeafes, and need not here be defcribed, further than by obferving, that they chiefly tend to the prefervation of a pure air, by keeping the patients, and the apartments in

O

which

which they lie, as clean as poffible, and by expeditioufly removing the infectious fæces to a proper diftance.

ALL practitioners feem agreed, that vomits are the medicines firft indicated in this difeafe: The naufea and fpontaneous difcharge of bilious matters from the ftomach, and the febrile ftate of the body in the commencement of this difeafe, clearly point out the propriety of emetics; but I here confider them as operating in full dofes, and not in fmall quantities, as will be prefently defcribed.

WITH refpect to bleeding, it has been formerly efteemed a fort of maxim, that " *Dyfenteria quâ dyfenteria, venæfectionem indicat nunquam;*" but, like all other general rules, this will admit of exception, even in the contagious dyfentery of hot climates, which is not unfrequently in the beginning attended with fome inflammatory fymptoms ‡.---- The pulfe, heat, &c. and not the tormina or gripings, afford the trueft indication for the ufe of this remedy; for the pain of the bowels feems generally to depend more on fpafm, and an increafed periftaltic motion, than on any confiderable degree of inflammation.

To remove this fpafm, which is the principal caufe and fupport of the difeafe, no means have yet been found fo univerfally beneficial as the ufe of *laxatives.*   UNDER

‡ PRINGLE, p. 236 ——CLEGHORN Dif. *Minorca.*——MONRO'S Dif. Army, p. 6.——LIND'S Dif. hot Clim. p. 249.——ZIMMERMANN, p. 179.

UNDER this head, perhaps, fmall dofes of emetics are to be confidered, though it is probable they have here, as in fever, a double action, affecting both the bowels and the fkin *.----Ipecacuanha in particular has been celebrated for its antidyfenteric virtues, and is unqueftionably one of the beft medicines; but, confidered as a purgative, it is too limited in its operation, and fhould not be given till others of a more active though mild nature have been employed; fuch as, the purging falts, tamarinds, and cr. tartar, &c. Upon the repeated ufe of fuch gentle purges during the firft ftage of the difeafe, principally depends our future fuccefs †; but regard muft always be had to the ftrength of the patient, and his capacity for bearing evacuations.

To enter into a full detail of the various other modes of practice, and medicines made ufe of in the cure of dyfentery, would be a fubject for a much larger work than the prefent one; and therefore, omitting the confideration of diluents, demulcents, aftringents, bark, clyfters, &c, all of them in their proper place remedies of great efficacy and importance, I fhall conclude the cure of dyfentery by a remark or two on the *diaphoretic* practice, and the ufe of opiates.

SOME

---

* See PRINGLE.

† Purgantia fere fola medicamenta funt quæ hodie ad dyfenteriam depellendam neceffaria exiftimantur.————WARDROP *de Dyf. Malig.*

Vide alfo ZIMMERMANN, PRINGLE, MONRO, &c. &c. who trufted the cure of dyfentery chiefly to the ufe of evacuants.

SOME authors have denied the exiftence of fever in dyfentery; but it would feem that they have never met with the
epidemic kind: for the contrary has been almoft univerfally
obferved, and SYDENHAM confidered it as a fever turned
inwards upon the bowels.   It is from hence, I prefume,
and from the effects of cold air, in conftringing the furface, and determining to the bowels, that the diaphoretic
indication has been drawn.   Experience has fufficiently
demonftrated the good effects of this practice in cold climates, where the circumftances indicating it prevail in a
greater degree; but in the Weft-Indies, I apprehend it is
neceffary to put fome reftrictions upon it.----There is no
means of preferving a pure air about the patient, but by a
free expofition to the breeze, which will always have the
effect of counteracting the operation of fweating medicines,
or endanger the bringing on of a greater degree of fpafm.
Forcible remedies of this fort fhould therefore be avoided;
but, as a gentle moifture, kept up conftantly upon the fkin,
ferves greatly to diminifh the impetus upon the bowels, and
alleviate the tormina, the ufe of a flannel fhirt may be of
great utility, as this defends the patient from the action of
the air, which is of neceffity admitted for carrying off the
contagious effluvia.---Many other remarks might be made
on this fubject, but I proceed to opiates *.

IT

---

* To the diaphoretic method of cure may perhaps be referred the practice
principally followed at St. Lucia, which confifted in giving antimonials with
opium.——*Vide* ROLLO's *dif. of army at St. Lucia.*

IT was formerly thought, the violent pains and inceſſant motions, could only be mitigated by the uſe of opium; but experience teaches, that whatever temporary relief opiates may afford, they ultimately do harm, by increaſing the very ſymptoms they are intended to remove †. More benefit is derived in the beginning of this diſeaſe from laxatives, diluents, and fomentations; but, notwithſtanding the general complaint of the inefficacy and hurtful qualities of opium, there is no practitioner that can do without it:--it is ſometimes abſolutely neceſſary as a palliative, till other medicines arrive at their effects; and in the latter ſtage, after the full uſe of evacuations, it will prove the beſt means of allaying irritability ‡.

HAVING now, in as conciſe a manner as I have been able, pointed out ſome of the moſt eſſential circumſtances inducing and relating to the diſeaſes of the troops at SAN JUAN, I have only to implore the candour of my readers, to judge as favourably as they can of ſo imperfect a publication.

---

† Almoſt all authors are agreed, in thinking opium hurtful in the beginning of this diſeaſe.————See ZIMMERMAN, PRINGLE, MONRO, TRALLER, DEGNER; MOSELEY's *Treatiſe on the Dyſentery of the* Weſt Indies.

‡ WARDROP.

www.ingramcontent.com/pod-product-compliance
Lightning Source LLC
Chambersburg PA
CBHW021526090426
42739CB00007B/793